How to Avoid Brain Aging Dementia – Memory Loss

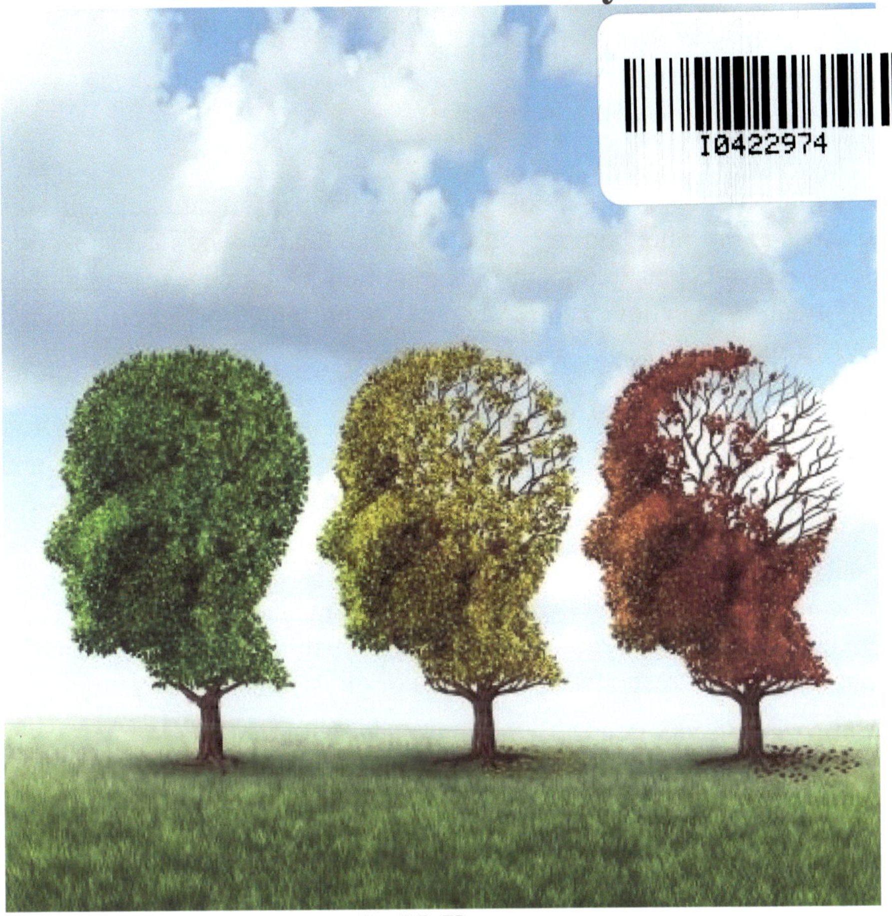

By M. Usman
Health Learning Series
Mendon Cottage Books

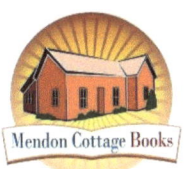

JD-Biz Publishing

Disclaimer

The information is this book is provided for informational purposes only. It is not intended to be used and medical advice or a substitute for proper medical treatment by a qualified health care provider. The information is believed to be accurate as presented based on research by the author.

The contents have not been evaluated by the U.S. Food and Drug Administration or any other Government or Health Organization and the contents in this book are not to be used to treat cure or prevent disease.

The author or publisher are not responsible for the use or safety of any diet, procedure or treatment mentioned in this book. The author or publisher is not responsible for errors or omissions that may exist.

Warning

The Book is for informational purposes only and before taking on any diet, treatment or medical procedure it is recommended to consult with your primary care provider.

Our books are available at

1. Amazon.com
2. Barnes and Noble
3. Itunes
4. Kobo
5. Smashwords
6. Google Play Books

Table of Contents

Introduction

Is increasing age withering the performance of your brain? Are you clueless how to avoid the side effects of aging on your brain health? Is your aging brain ruining your life? No matter how many problems you have faced because of your increasing age, "How to avoid brain aging?" gives you a quick review of all the dos and don'ts for a successful brain aging.

Each chapter of this book gives you a deep insight to the basic causes of brain aging and helps answer your basic question: "How to avoid brain aging?"

Following the guidelines regarding life style changes, eating habits, social interactions and habits to avoid, you can overcome the problem of brain aging in a quick and effective manner and can lead a healthy and active life.

Section one: How human brain works?

Human brain is the center of all our activities. Human brain is like a puzzle, the complexity of which is beyond comprehension.

Human brain is truly a miracle of nature. It's like a super computer that processes millions of information each second with us even knowing. It starts functioning form the time of birth and continues to work till death. It works 24 hours a day, 7 days a week without taking rest for even a single second. All our routine activates like reading a novel, listening to a song, kicking a football, solving a mathematical problem, watching TV, using computer or mobile etc. are interpreted in our brain in the form chemical and electrical changes that travel from one neuron to another. These neurons are like keys of a piano, when played in a particular sequence produce the symphony of life.

A neuron or a nerve cell is the basic structural and functional unit of human brain. Human brain is made of several billion of such neurons. These neurons are not just scattered in the brain, but are connected with each other through an extremely complex and intricate network of connections known as "synapses". These synapses are like a railway station, where different impulses are relayed and are then issued towards their target destination. Impulses are transmitted within a neuron in the form a minute "electrical current". When this current reaches the synapse, it causes the release of chemical substances known as "neurotransmitters" within the synapse. These chemicals produce a current in the preceding neurons. This transmission of signals from one neuron to another is like the runners of a "relay race", in which one runner passes the relay to his successive partner.

These impulses are either excitatory or inhibitory in nature leading to the activation or inhibition of successive neurons.

An event, accident or a particular activity makes way to our memory when it elicits a particular useful response in our brain. Like all other parts of human body, human brain works on the principal of "use it or lose it". If a particular experience elicits a useful response in a person, it is stored in the storage bin of our brain. But, if the response doesn't elicit such response, this information is discarded. That's why, almost 99% of the information we gather through reading, listening or watching is discarded by our brain. Only 1% of the useful information makes way to the storage bins of human brain.

What is brain aging?

Aging is an inevitable process that affects all organs of human body. Aging dements the efficiency, structure and function of human brain. It's the basic reason of forgetfulness and decreased mental activity experienced by a person as he ages. The breakdown of old neurons and formation of new ones is perfectly balanced in a normal individual i.e. the total number of neurons that degrade is equal to the total number of new neurons that grow. However, several experimental studies have shown that the rate of neuronal degradation increases several folds as a person ages. This increased rate of neuron break down was thought to be the basic culprit of brain aging. However, recent studies have shown that the rate of neuron regeneration is sufficient enough to support the normal brain activity.

So, a question arises in mind "what is the basic cause of brain aging?" This is a burning question in all the scientific communities and efforts are being made to present the most logical explanation for the basic cause of brain aging. The results of several researches indicate that brain aging is a combined effect of several factors like:

- The increased rate of neuronal break down definitely has a part in brain aging.
- The total number of neuronal synapses decreases significantly as a person ages. Decreased number of synapses, in turn, causes slowing of communication between neurons.
- Aging dements the plasticity of neurons i.e. the ability of neurons to adapt to life experiences. It decreases the learning and thinking ability of elderly persons.
- Several changes are observed in the physical structure of human brain as age progresses. Previously, only "grey matter" was considered to be the functional part of human brain. "White matter", on the other hand, was just considered to be a supportive part of brain. However, advancement in studies has disclosed the importance of white matter. White matter is made of neurons fibers and is thus necessary in the transmission of electrical impulses. There is a significant decrease in the volume of white matter in elderly persons. Shrinkage of white matter means impaired transmission of electrical impulses and decreased activity of brain. The basic causes of this shrinkage are still unclear.

How to avoid brain aging?

Brain aging is an inevitable process. There are several side effects of brain aging, like:

- Forgetfulness.

- Decreased sense of time, space and person.
- Decreased attention.
- Inability to focus on the given task.
- Decreased ability to learn new things.
- Decreased ability to hand parallel tasks.
- Inability to put together tiny bits of information to reach to a logical solution.
- Inability to make critical decision.
- Increased stress and anxiety.

Scientists have observed that the mental performance of some elderly individuals is far better than the other individuals of same age group. It's believed that different factors that help avoid the side effects of brain aging include:

- Those individuals that are in the habit of doing regular exercise and physical activities are less prone to the side effects of brain aging. Mild physical activities like jogging, gardening, walking etc. help a lot in improving brain function.
- Those people that try to use their brain in learning new things stay mentally active even in the late stages of their life. An idle life style speeds up the damaging effects of brain aging.
- People that are involved in social activities and are better tied to their friends and families remain healthy mentally and physically.
- The way of thinking is a key factor that can either improve or dement the activity of human brain. Continuous stress has deleterious effects on brain health.

- Similarly, those individuals that avoided alcohol, smoking, drugs and excessive use of medicines and supplements were found to be healthier than the others.

In short, all these petty changes are the key factors that distinguish among the individuals of a community. Minor changes in your life style can greatly enhance your brain activity.

Section two: What to do, to avoid brain aging

Regular exercise

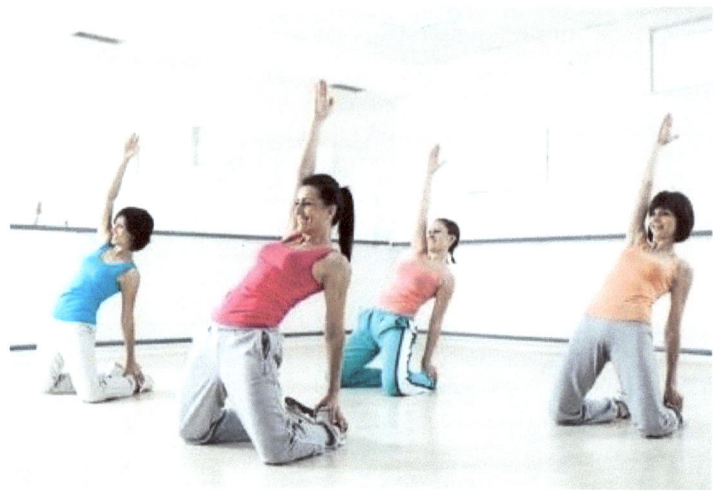

It's a general observation that what is good for the health of our body is good for our brain as well. Exercise doesn't mean that you have to run in a marathon race. Mild physical activities like brisk walking, jogging, playing a game like golf or simple exercise can help a lot in improving the health of your brain and reducing the chances of several brain disorders like Alzheimer's disease. 30 minutes of such activities two or three times a week are sufficient for an individual. Those physical activities are particularly very beneficial that involve learning of new stuff like aerobics and a new type of dance.

A question might come to mind "How exercise and physical activities help avoid the side effects of brain aging?" The beneficial effects of exercise on brain health are because of its ability to bring about following changes in the human body:

- Aging suppresses the activity of human brain because it makes the human brain sluggish and increases the response time to a stimulus. This increase in the response time of neurons is because of decreased plasticity of neurons. As the result, a person is unable to think properly and make quick decision. Recent brain imaging techniques have shown that regular exercise and physical activities help improve the neuronal connection and thus help improve the plasticity of neuronal synapses.
- Grey matter is the basic functional part of human brain that contains all the nerve bodies. Regular exercise helps prevent the shrinkage of grey matter and thus help improve the brain function.
- Regular exercise increases the rate of formation of new neurons. A process known as "neurogenesis". Several experiments performed on

  laboratory animals have shown that those rats that were involved in some kinds of physical activities had an improved level of brain activity and they were able to find a way out of a maze much more quickly as compared to those rats that weren't involved in such activities.
- Regular exercise and physical activities promote the production of several "nerve growth factors". These factors promote the process of neurogeneis.

- Regular exercise helps improve the flow of blood to the brain. Increase in the supply of blood, in turn, improves the supply of oxygen and nutrients to brain and helps the clearing of waste products from brain matrix.

- Regular exercise and physical activities provide an effective retreat from daily routine and all the tension related with it. In this way, exercise also helps relieve tension and anxiety.

Healthy diet

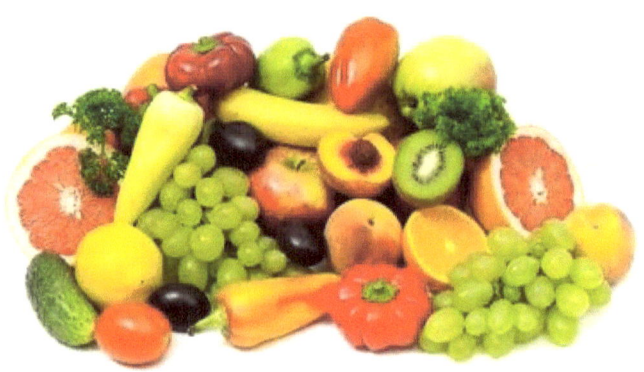

A balanced and healthy diet is the basic requirement for a healthy brain. The basic reason of brain aging, in most of the cases, is poor nutrition that is unable to supply the essential nutrients to brain. Like any other part of human body, human brain requires sufficient supply of carbohydrates, proteins, vitamins and minerals to perform its activities in an effective manner. All these components of a healthy diet help improve the structure and performance of human brain. The deficiency of these nutrients can also lead to serious mental complication. A brain healthy diet is derived from following food groups:

- Vegetables and fruits: Colorful fruits and vegetables are naturally rich in all the vitamins and minerals that are required for normal brain activity. All vegetables and fruits are rich in carbohydrates and proteins but are low in cholesterol. Low level of cholesterol not only helps decrease the chances of brain hemorrhage but also decrease the chances of cardiovascular events like heart failure and high blood pressure. Moreover, this food group is rich in fibers that help improve the absorption of minerals and vitamins.

- Milk: Milk and all the dairy products are a rich source of calcium. Calcium is the basic mineral required for normal nerve transmission. Moreover, dairy products are rich in "good fats" that are essential for brain function.

- Anti-oxidants: Anti-oxidants include several fat soluble vitamins like vitamin A, C, D and E. These vitamins are naturally present in sources like egg, liver, green leafy vegetables and meat. Anti-oxidants are extremely beneficial because they decrease the production of "reactive oxygen species (ROS)". ROS inflict significant damage to the structure of neurons and thus exterminate their normal activity. Use of multi-vitamins is usually recommended if the normal diet is poor in vitamin content.

- Omega-3 fatty acids: This group includes members like linoleic acid, linolenic acid and arachadonic acid. These fatty acids are mainly present in sea food. These "good fats" help improve brain function in following manner:
  - These fats help reduce the production of reactive oxygen species (ROS) and damage inflicted by them.
  - These fats help stabilize the structure of neurons.
  - These fatty acids are necessary for the development of glaial cells. Glail cells are the basic supportive cells of human brain that help protect and provide nutrition to the neurons.

- Vitamins: A healthy brain carves and requires the supply of vitamins. Several vitamins help improve function of brain:
  - Folic acid is required for normal brain function.
  - Vitamin B12, vitamin B6 and other B complex are the integral component of several neurons that help provide energy required for brain function.
  - Vitamin D, E and A is anti-oxidant.

- Carbohydrates: Human brain can't metabolize fats for the generation of energy. It depends on second to second supply of carbohydrates for meeting its energy requirements. So, eating a diet rich in carbohydrates help improve brain function.

Healthy social interactions

Healthy social interactions are the basic pre-requisite required to avoid brain aging. Activates or gatherings that involve you interacting with your friends, neighbors and family are very beneficial in improving the cognitive abilities of your brain. Healthy social interactions include dance parties, playing card or golf with your friends, going into weddings or birthday parties, traveling with friends etc.

Humans are a civilized species. Humans colonized the land and started living in groups and clans. That's how human beings are supposed to live. Human beings live in groups, live and interact with each other. Isolation brings nothing but utter eradication of brain function. Isolation promotes illness of brain and anti-social behaviors in a person. It increases the level of stress and anxiety and totally impairs the learning and thinking abilities of a person.

A better social interaction helps improve brain function and helps avoid aging of brain in following manner:

- Better social interactions promote the cognitive functions of brain.
- It soothes the mind and helps a person think properly.
- It helps a person concentrate on a given task.
- Social interactions are particularly very beneficial in promoting brain health because it is a common observation that the things we learn in a group are better remembered by our brain as compared to those things that a person learns alone.
- It gives one with an opportunity to share his or her problems with his or her friends and family. Sharing decreases the level of stress and anxiety- the basic reason of brain aging.

- It helps a person learn from the experiences of his friends and relatives.
- It helps a person broaden his mind and helps him learn new things and new experiences.
- Healthy social interactions induce a sense of responsibility in a person and help him work as a unit with his companions. In this way, social interactions bless a person with good mood and healthy mind.

Improve your brain potential

Several studies have proved that individuals that are involved in some sort of mental activity are less prone to the harmful effects of aging and brain illnesses.

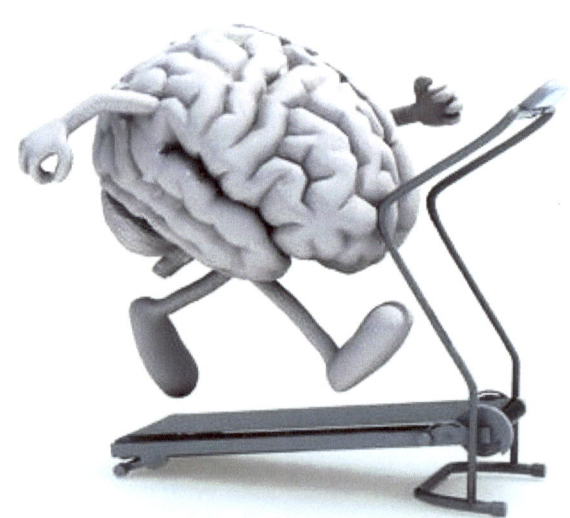

According to a report published by "Journal of American medical association", cognitive training programs conducted on elderly people improved their cognition, learning and thinking abilities.

Cognitive training programs help a person make better use of his or her brain in an effective manner. It helps a person do his daily activities in a proficient way. But what is cognitive training? Cognitive training is a program designed to improve the potential of human brain. Such training of brain helps improve the quantity and plasticity of neuronal synapses. Thus, help decrease the response time to a particular stimulus. Such training programs help improve the function of human brain on three different fronts:

- Memory: Anything useful, that elicits the brain centers is stored in the memory bins of brain. This part of cognitive training program involves simple tricks that help a person memorize things like text materials, grocery items, color combinations, number combinations and main idea of a novel or story.

- Reasoning skills: This part of cognitive training helps sharpen brain skills including solving a mathematical problems, putting together bits of information to reach to a logical goal, filling out a order sheet or solving a puzzle or maze etc.

- Response time of brain: This part of training is focused on improving the response time of brain. It can help a person perform daily activities like looking up a phone number in list, looking up for an individual on a contact list or finding information on a bottle of medicine.

Section three: Avoid these to avoid brain aging

Alcohol intake

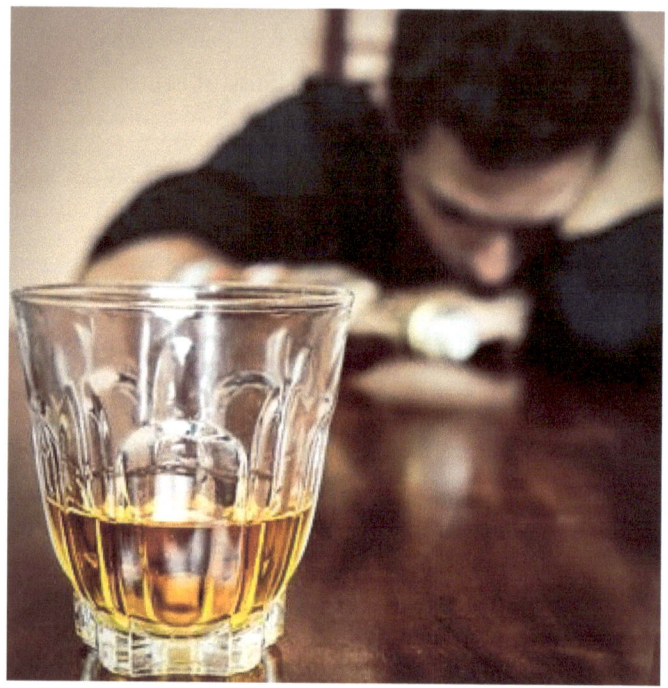

The intake of alcohol has both immediate and long term effects on brain health. The immediate effects of alcohol consumption on brain health include:

- Impaired thinking.
- Inability to make decisions.
- Inability to focus on a particular task.
- Anxiety.
- Inability to think logically.

- Sluggishness of mental activity.
- Blurring of vision.
- Slurring of speech.

All these effects of alcohol consumption are temporary and wither as soon as the drinking is discontinued.

The side effects of alcohol intake vary from simple symptoms like slip of memory to serious and permanent damage of brain. Several factors determine the extent of damage of alcohol on brain health:

- The frequency and quantity of alcohol intake.
- For how long the person has been drinking.
- One's general state of health since the side effects of alcohol damage are more prominent when a person has poor health.
- Age, family history and gender of an individual.

The long term side effects of alcohol intake include:

- Chronic alcohol intake produces deficiency of an essential vitamin known as "thiamine". Thiamine is essentially required for the proper functioning of brain. It is also required for the energy generation in body. Deficiency of thiamine produces a mental disorder known as "Wernicke-Korsakoff's syndrome".

- Prolong intake of alcohol produces serious disturbance in the normal sleep-wake cycle of human body. It produces insomnia, anxiety and depression. All these factors suppress the development of human brain.

- Intake of alcohol increase the chances of short term as well and long term memory loss.
- It greatly increases the chances of mental disorders like Alzheimer's disease.

So, the use of alcohol should be totally avoided if you want to avoid brain aging.

Drug abuse

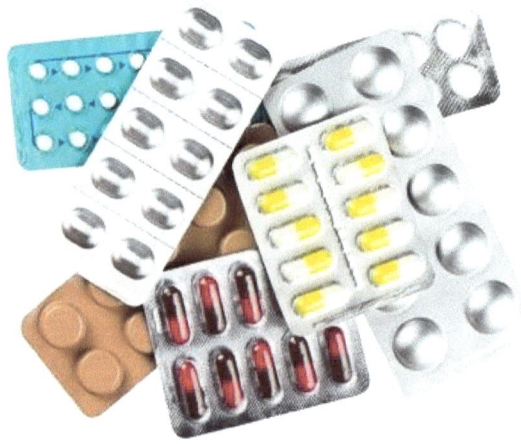

The abuse of drugs has damaging effects on the mental and physical health of an individual. Drugs alter the way in which human brain works. Different drugs that mutilate the normal brain function include:

- Heroine.
- Cocaine.
- Morphine.
- Tranquilizers.

- Amphetamines.
- Barbiturates.
- Ephedrine.
- Opiates.
- Hypnotics.

Most of the people fall for these drugs because these drugs excite the "reward center" of human brain. When this center of human brain is activated, brain releases a large amount of a hormone known as "dopamine" in the circulation. When this hormone acts on the nerve synapses it causes a feeling of light headedness, pain suppression, euphoria, pleasure and relief. But, the excessive and chronic release of this hormone causes brain damage.

Different addictive drugs with their mode of action on human brain are listed as follows:

- Hallucinogenic drugs: Lysergic acid diethylamide, which goes by the street name of LSD, is the prototypic drug of this family. These drugs produce alerted sense of time, "spiritual experiences", relaxation and light headedness. However, the use of LSD can induce mental disorders like schizophrenia and mental depression.

- Stimulatory drugs: This group includes drugs like amphetamines, cocaine, ephedrine and phenylephrine. These drugs either decrease the reuptake of norepinephrine and dopamine from neuronal synapse or increase the release of dopamine and norepinephrine from neurons. As, the result, the total quantity of these neurotransmitters in the neuronal synapse increases and produce effects like euphoria and increased attention to a given task. However, the side effects include extensive mood swings, anorexia, apathy, insomnia and anxiety.

- Depressant drugs: Alcohol, heroine and morphine are the basic prototypic drugs of this group. These drugs act by the release of several "inhibitory neurotransmitters" that depress the level of brain activity. The use of these drugs produce signs like light headedness, relief of pain, relaxation and sleep. However, the prolong use of these drugs produce a phenomenon of "dependence". In this condition, the person remains intoxicated as long as he is taking these drugs. But, when he stops taking the drugs, it produces conditions like delirium, intense pain, tremors, anxiety and impaired thinking.

So, the use of these drugs should be avoided as the use of these drugs not only impairs the normal functioning of human brain but also increases the chances of severe mental illness.

Inadequate sleep

Human body is not a machine. It needs proper rest for proper mental and physical activities. Adequate sleep helps improve brain health:

- Sleep promotes the production of several hormones that help in the development of new neurons.
- Sleep helps conserve energy.

- It helps in the consolidation of memory.
- It helps improve the cognitive abilities of brain.

Inadequate sleep is one of the basic problems faced by people as they age. The side effects of inadequate sleep include:

- Drowsiness impairs brain functions.
- Inadequate sleep makes a person lethargic.
- It impairs one's thinking ability and prevents him to make decisions.
- Improper sleep promotes the death of neurons.

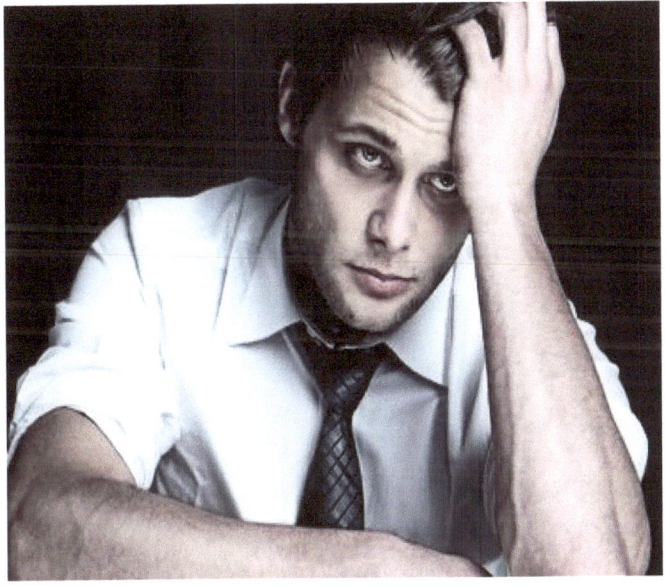

So, proper sleep is one of the basic pre-requisites required to avoid aging of human brain. If you are suffering from insomnia or if you complain of improper quantity and quality of sleep then following are some tips for you to promote normal sleep:

- Try to fix a "go to bed" and "get up" time.

- Consume lesser fluids before going to bed.

- Avoid heavy meals for at least 1-2 hours before going to bed.

- Avoid excessive intake of caffeine and alcohol since these compounds impair normal sleep-wake cycle.

- Nicotine present in cigarette prevents normal sleep. So, avoid cigarette smoking.

- Regular sleep promotes the supply of blood to all parts of body and helps improve the quality as well as the quantity of sleep.

- Take hot bath before going to bed.

- Select a room or place that has least public interference.

- Select a room with least noise.

- Adjust the light in the room as you sleep.

- Adjust the room temperature.

- Choose a bed or mattress which is comfortable for you.

Stress

Stress is a double edged sword as far the activity of human brain is concerned. Acute stress, the kind of stress that we experience during an accident or during our exams etc, can actually help improve the function of human brain in following manner:

- Human brain has the ability to adapt to the surrounding conditions. As we face an eminent threat or danger, the level of stress increases the generalized brain activity and helps us think of the best solution in shortest time possible.

- Stress increases the supply of sugar to brain that helps brain to get extra energy for increased activity.

- It increases the supply of blood to brain and helps supply extra oxygen to the brain.

- Acute stress causes the release of hormones known as "glucocorticoides". These hormones help in the consolidation of memory. That's why accidents or events related with some kind of stress of emergency are remembered throughout the entire life.

However, the chronic exposure of human brain to high levels of glucocorticoids, as seen in prolonged stress, inflict serious damage to mental health, promote brain aging and impair the cognitive abilities of human brain.

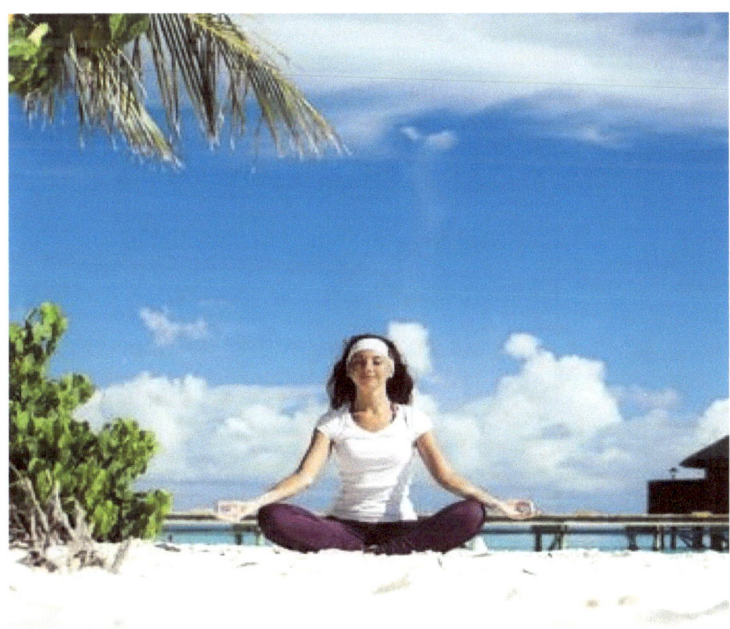

So, stress management is one of the most effective methods to avoid brain aging. Several methods can be used to avoid stress. Such methods include:

- Yoga: Yoga is one of the most effective methods that can be used for stress management. It helps reduce stress in following basic manner:
  - ✓ It improves the supply of blood to brain.
  - ✓ It helps clear mind and helps a person think clearly.
  - ✓ It helps relieve body pain and aches.
  - ✓ Meditation and yoga provide an effective retreat from your daily routine.
- Regular exercise: It is another effective method for stress management. It helps improve the supply of blood and nutrients to brain and helps improve the focus of an individual.
- Knowing your limits: In most of the cases, people face the problem of stress because they try to control the uncontrollable. For such people, here are some tips:
  - ✓ Don't try to control the uncontrollable.
  - ✓ Know your limits.
  - ✓ Don't burden yourself with extra work.
  - ✓ Don't blame yourself for everything happening around you.
  - ✓ Spare some time for yourself.
  - ✓ Add humor to your life.
  - ✓ A simple thing like ordinary smile can help a lot in solving a lot of problems.

- ✓ Try to forgive others.
- ✓ Avoid such people or such discussions that increase your stress or tension.
- ✓ Engage yourself in social activities.

So, stress management is very effective methods that can suppress the harmful effects of brain aging and can promote healthy effects on brain.

Health conditions

A long list of health complications can promote the degradation of human brain and can greatly speed up the process of brain aging. Such diseases include:

- High blood pressure: Hypertension is one of the major causes that promote negative changes in human brain. High blood pressure causes symptoms like throbbing headache, impaired thinking and confusion. Very high blood pressure can lead to increased chances of brain hemorrhage (stroke). It is one of the most common reasons of mental complication. It can cause both physical impairments and thinking abnormalities.
- Depression: It is another important cause of impaired mental function. It decreases cognition and induces dementia (forgetfulness).
- High cholesterol levels: Introduction of junk food and sedentary life as become the major health hazards for people of our age. It promotes the rise of cholesterol inside our body. This high level of cholesterol is deposited in the walls of blood vessels and

decreases the lumen of blood vessels. When there is a significant decrease in the lumen of blood vessels, these vessels burst and produce areas of brain damage. This condition is known as stroke. If stroke takes place in the areas of brain controlling the physical activities of body, it presents in the form of physical impairments like hemiplegia. Stroke in the sensory, memory bins or emotion centers produce irreversible damage in the learning abilities of a person.

- Degenerative diseases: There is a long list of brain disorders that preset themselves in the form of impaired physical functions, decreased learning abilities, decreased IQ and faster brain aging. The most common of such diseases include Huntington's disease, Parkinson's disease and Alzheimer's disease.

- Convulsive disorders: Such disorders include epilepsy and are characterized by impaired thinking and decreased cognition.

- Metabolic deriders: Impaired metabolism can lead to the accumulation of substances like glycogen and lipids. Such diseases include Tay sach's disease and Gaucher's disease. Such diseases are associated with increased rate of neuronal degradation and impaired learning.

- Infectious diseases: Several infectious diseases, like brain dementia, are also associated with impaired brain activity.

So, if you are facing any of these conditions then you should rush to your doctor and seek proper medical care because the final outcome of all these disorders is permanent brain damage.

Excessive use of medicines and supplements

All the medicines and supplements are recommended to cure a medical condition. But, the excessive use of medicines and supplements is very dangerous. Elderly people are particularly very prone to the harmful effects of medicines and supplements because their body systems and metabolic functions are seriously compromised. As the result, the drugs are neither properly metabolized nor are excreted from the body. So, it causes a significant increase in the blood levels of these drugs. Some drugs, after metabolism, are converted into toxic metabolites that not only affect the physical structure of brain but also alter the normal functioning of human brain.

The excessive use of vitamin supplements, similarly, can lead to a condition known as "hypervitaminosis". Vitamins, within a reasonable limit, are essential for brain function. But, when the levels of vitamins increase beyond safe limits, it produces side effects like dementia and impaired learning and thinking.

So, make sure you follow some points while using medicines and supplements:

- Never use a medicine or supplement without the prescription of your doctor. Since, self medication is one of the basic causes of drug related brain damage.
- Use the dosage as prescribed by the doctor.
- Use the medicines and supplements for as long the doctor has prescribed.
- If a drug produces some side effects, contact your clinician immediately.

- Tell your complete medicine and supplement history to your clinician upon checkup.

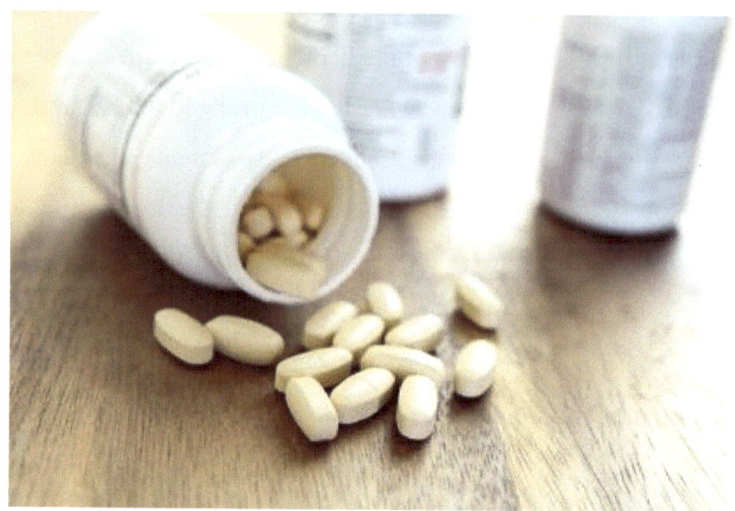

A quick review

Following is the checklist of habits that you should adopt in order to avoid brain aging:

- Exercise regularly.
- Always try to learn something new.
- Stay socially active.
- Always adopt a positive attitude.
- Never try to cross your limits as a human being.
- Try to avoid stress.
- Eat a diet rich in vegetables, fruits, anti-oxidants, vitamins and minerals.
- Get adequate sleep.
- Try to maintain normal blood cholesterol level.
- Manage your blood pressure.
- Consult your doctor if you face a medical condition.
- Avoid excessive intake of alcohol.
- Avoid smoking.
- Avoid self medication.
- Don't stay isolated.
- Never think that you are too old to learn something new.
- Never discuss those topics that aggravate your stress.
- Don't neglect any change in the health of your body and mind.
- Don't adopt a stagnant life style.

- Avoid getting into conversations with those people that leave you tensed and depressed.

Photo credits:

All Images Licensed by Fotolia.com

human brain on a running machine

© *fabioberti.it - Fotolia.com*

Vergesslicher Mann

© *damato - Fotolia.com*

Pretty woman doing yoga exercises on the tropical beach

© *Dmitry Sunagatov - Fotolia.com*

Women On Aerobic Class

© *luminastock - Fotolia.com*

fruits and vegetables isolated on a white background

© *SergheiVelusceac - Fotolia.com*

nk asleep man addicted to alcohol

© *kmiragaya - Fotolia.com*

Many tablets or pills

© *Sergey Lavrentev - Fotolia.com*

Stressed

© *lassedesignen - Fotolia.com*

Vitamins

© *JJAVA - Fotolia.com*

Author Bio

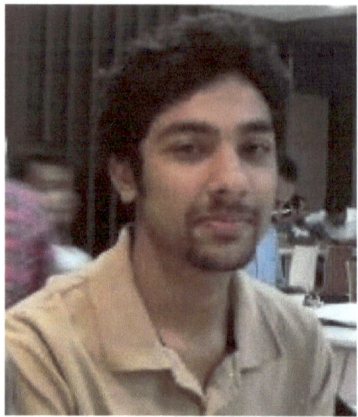

Muhammad Usman is a distinguished medical graduate of Allama iqbal medical college (AIMC). He is a professional writer who has been in the field for more than 4 years. During this time he has produced 10,000+ articles, blogs and eBooks on various niches related to diseases, health, fitness, nutrition and well being. He is a regular contributor to several journals related to medicine and surgery. He is the editor of several journals and newspapers.

Check out some of the other JD-Biz Publishing books

[Gardening Series on Amazon](#)

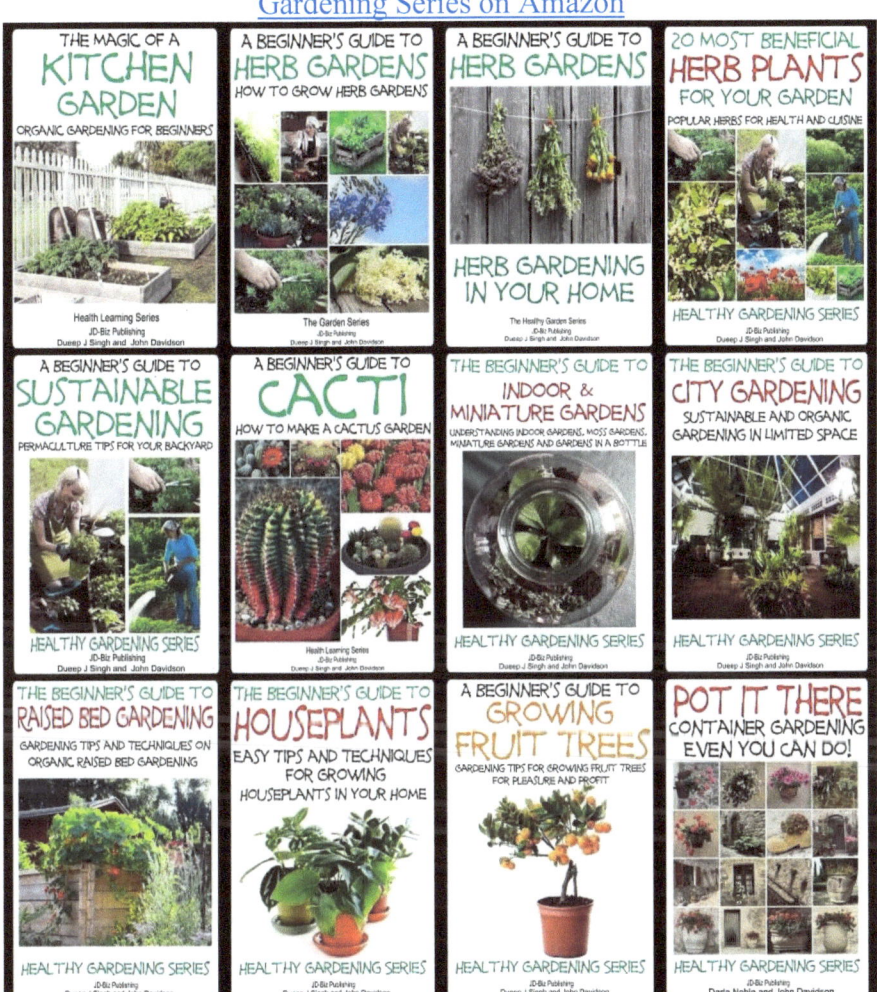

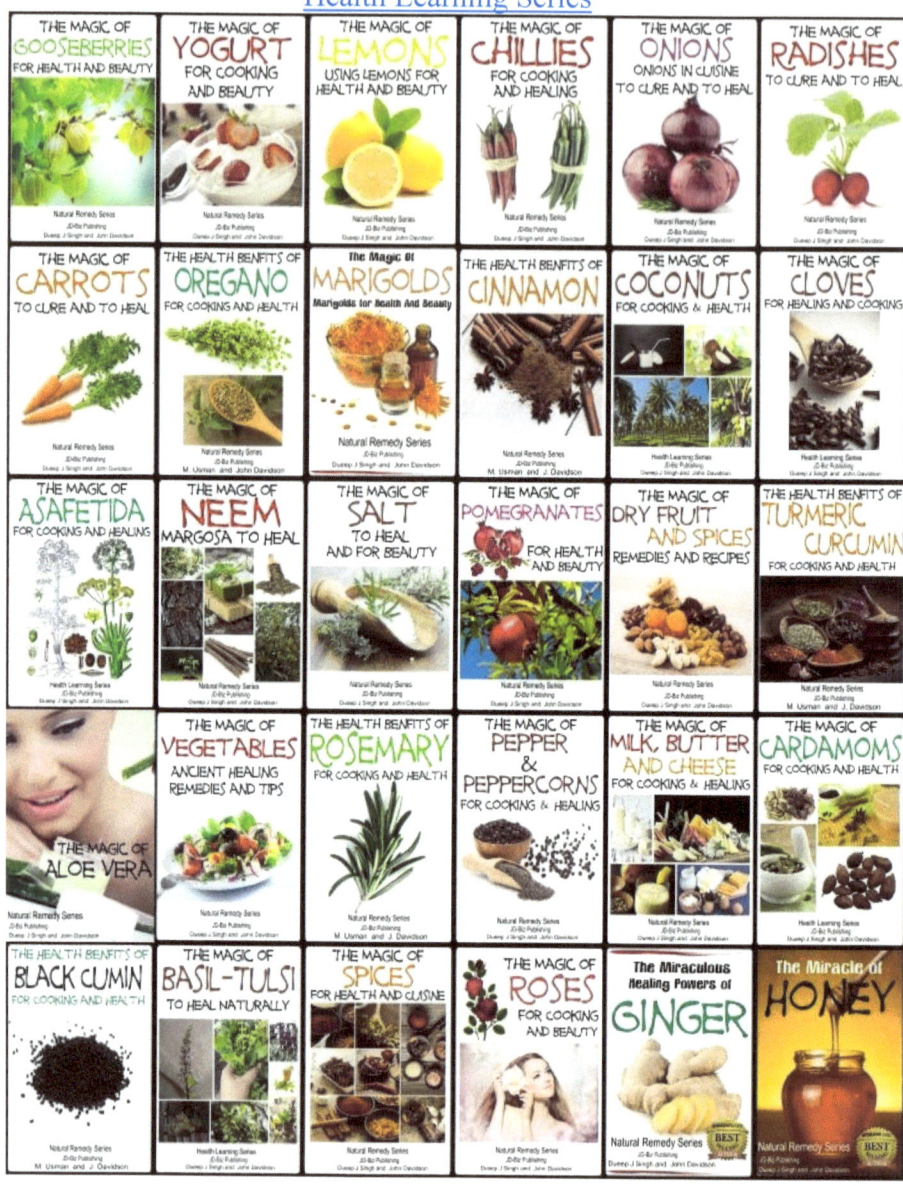

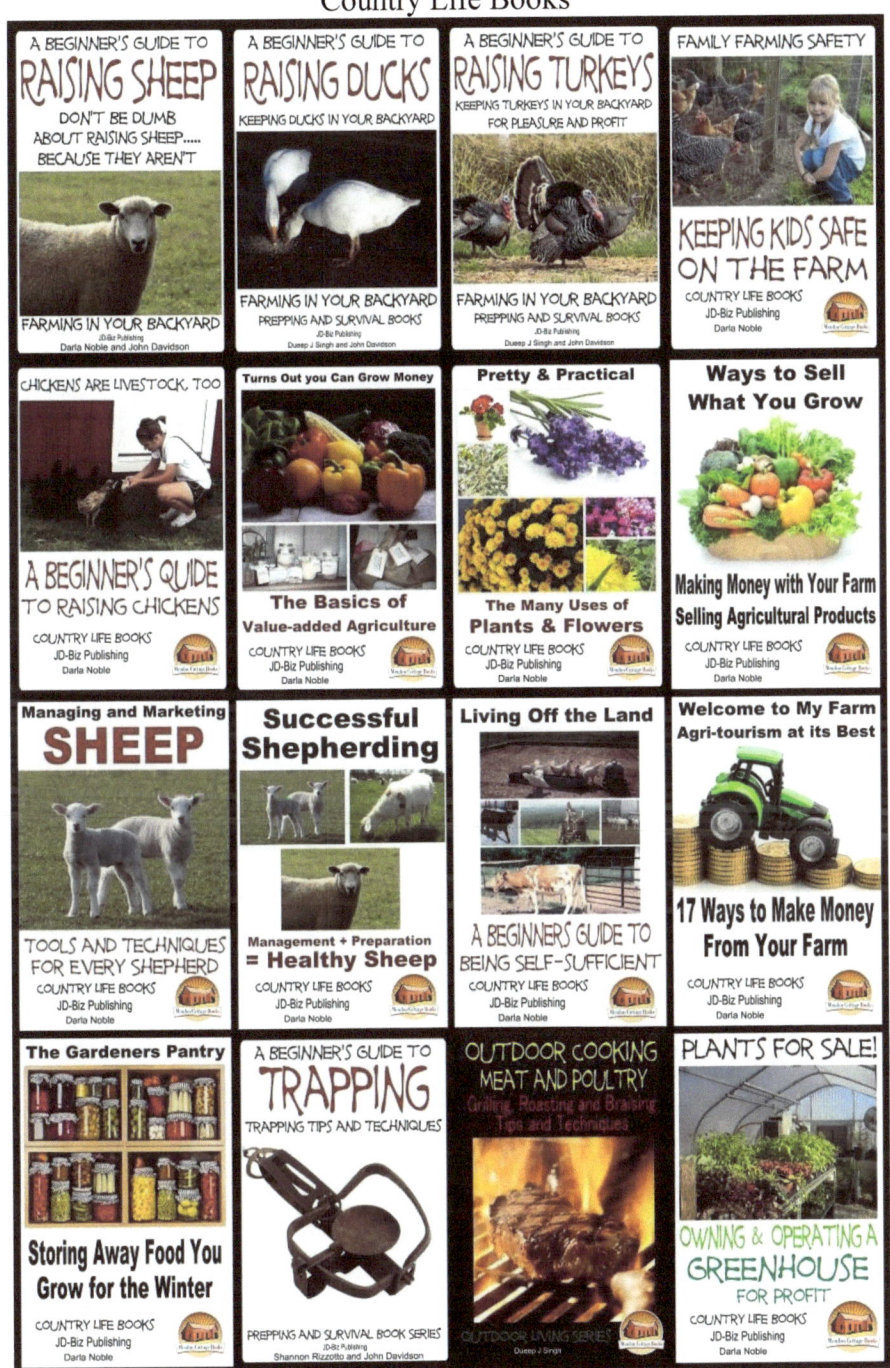

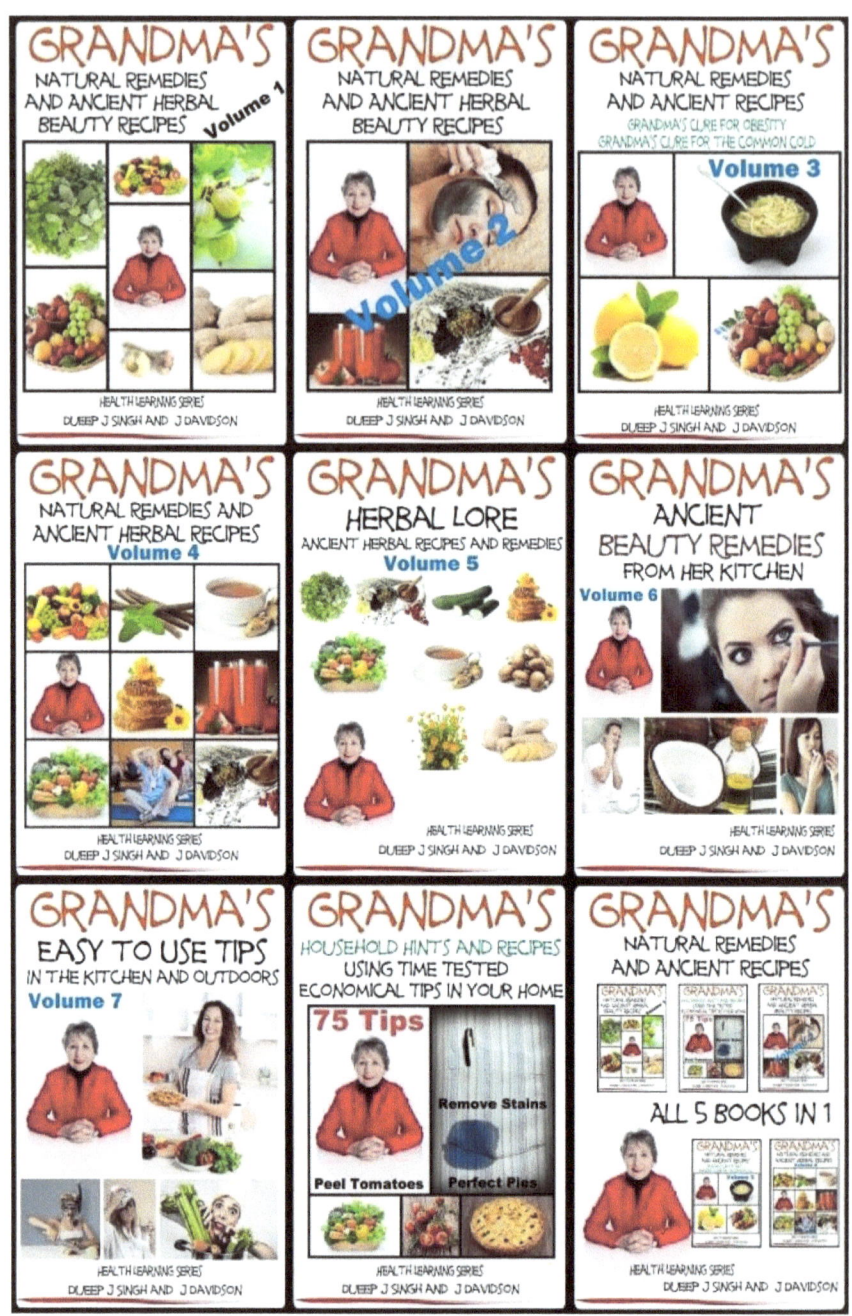

Health Learning Series

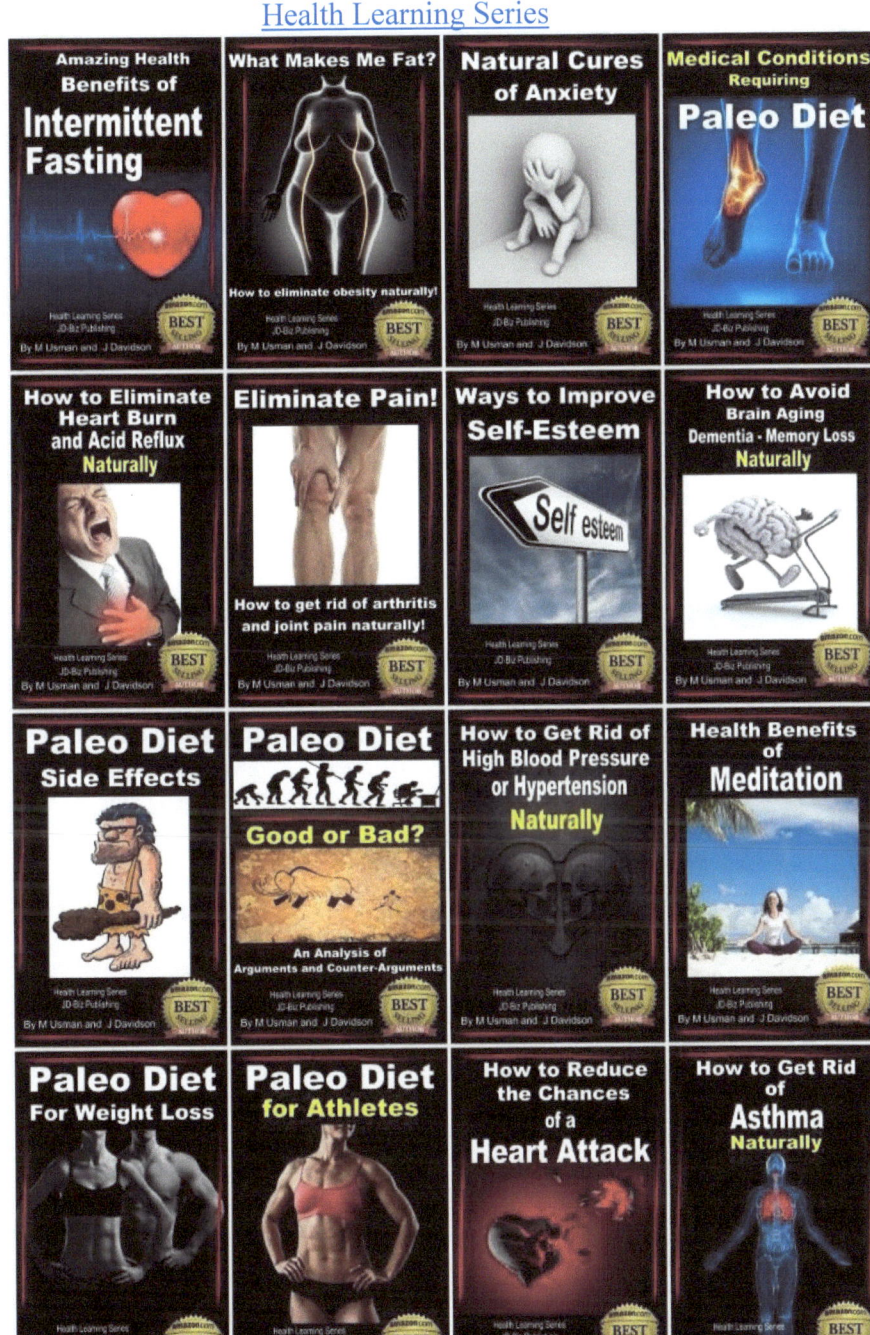

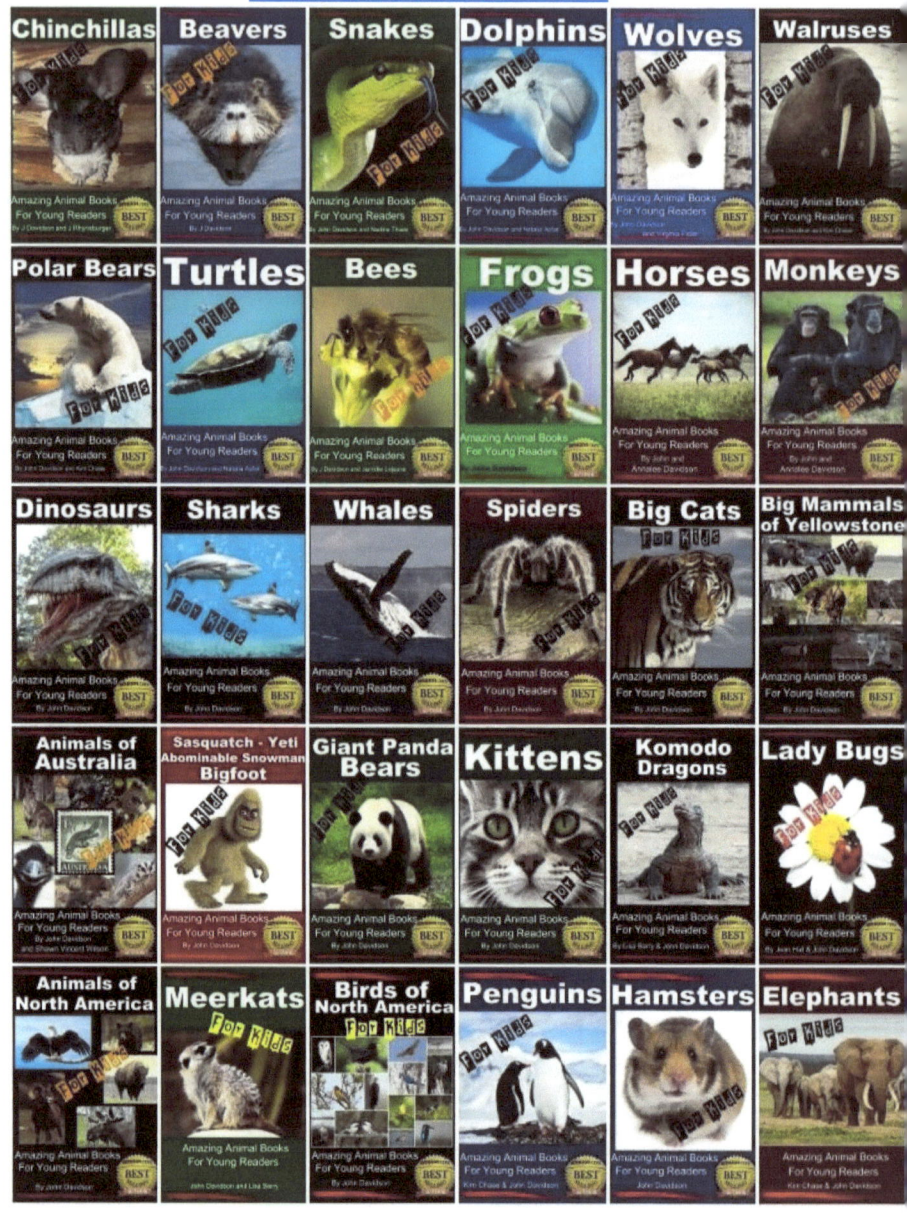

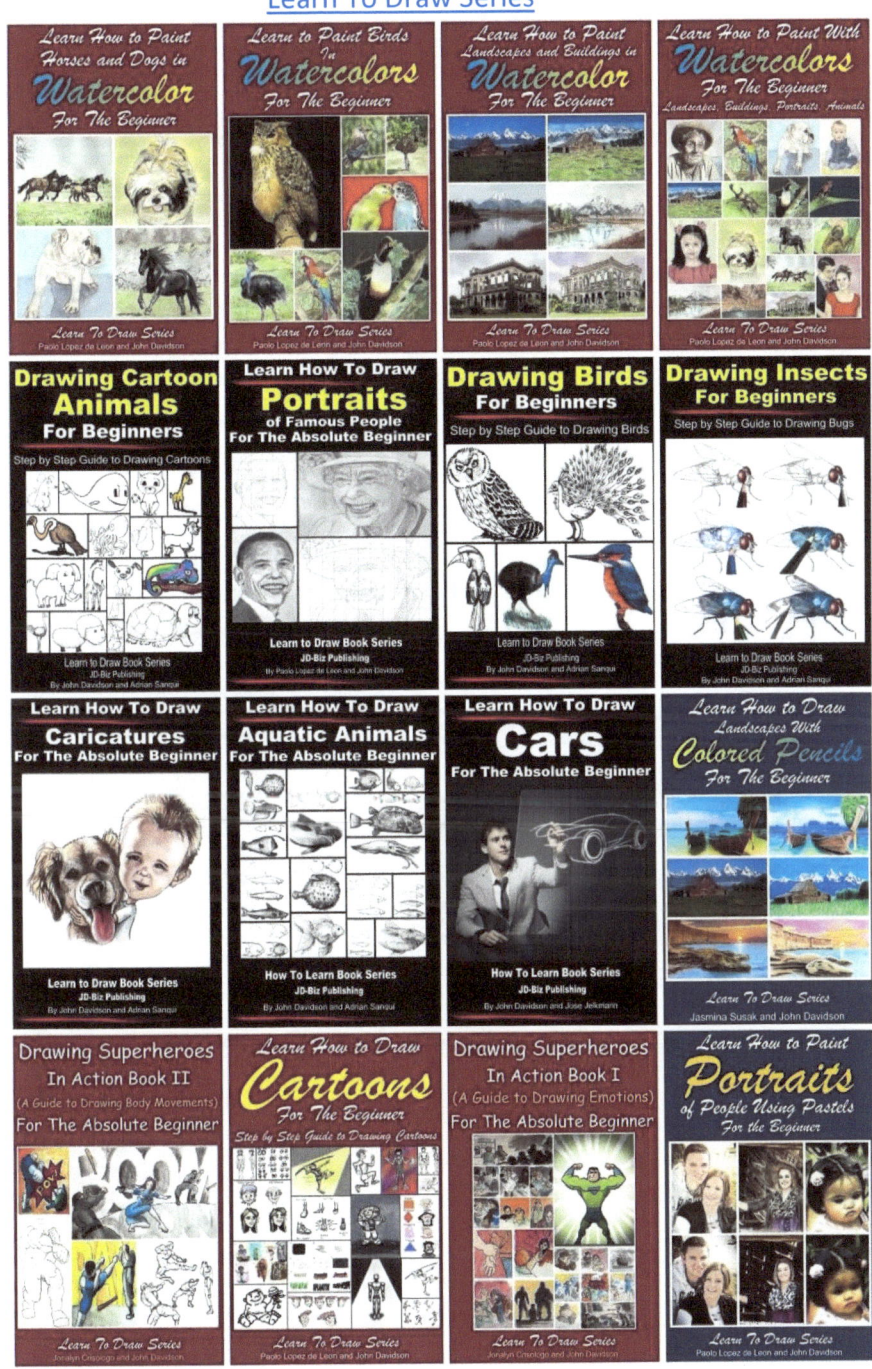

How to Build and Plan Books

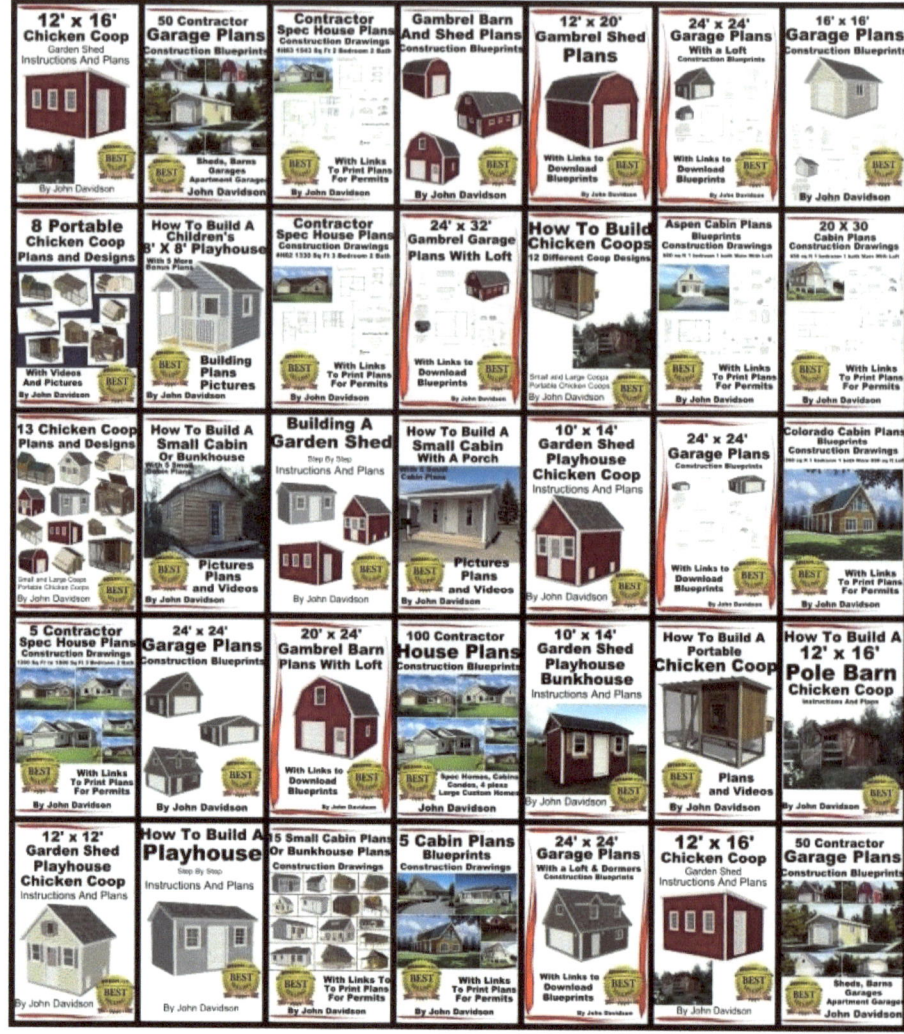

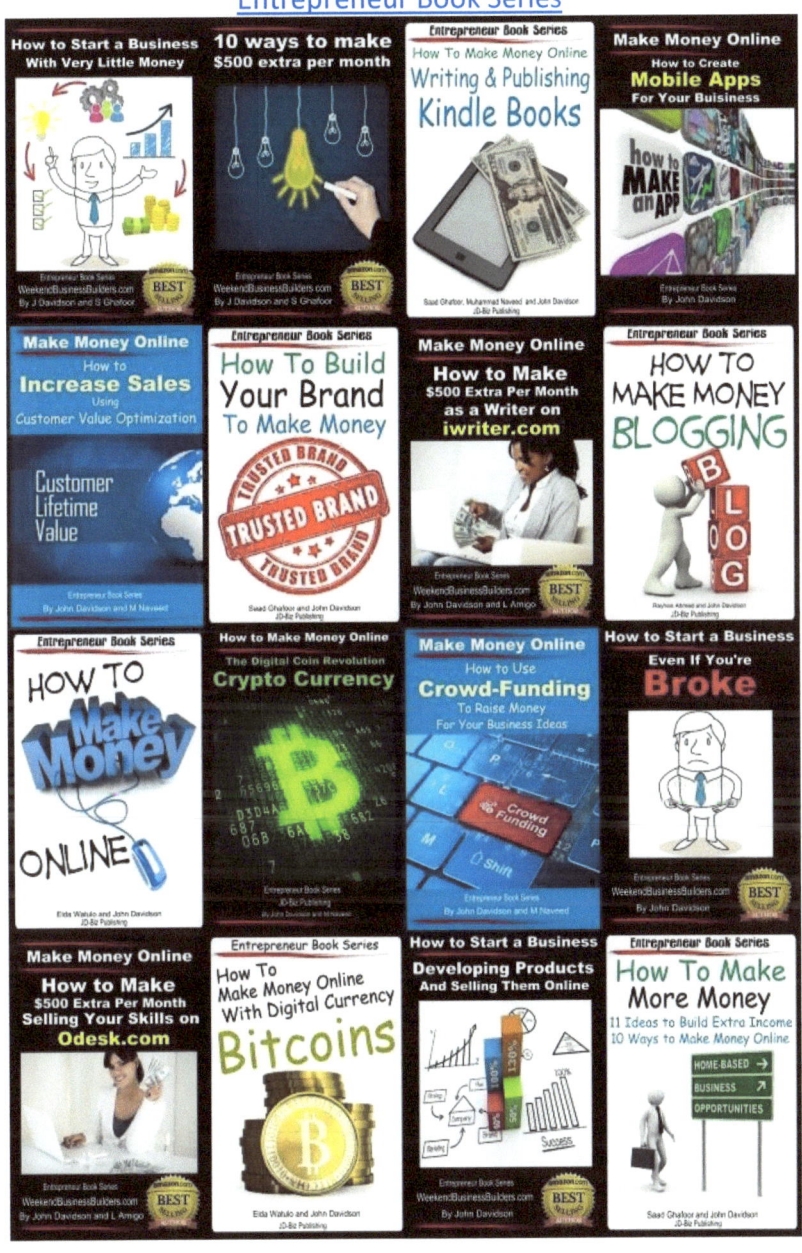

Our books are available at

1. Amazon.com
2. Barnes and Noble
3. Itunes
4. Kobo
5. Smashwords
6. Google Play Books

Download Free Books!
http://MendonCottageBooks.com

Publisher

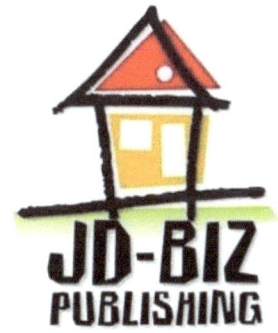

JD-Biz Corp

P O Box 374

Mendon, Utah 84325

http://www.jd-biz.com/

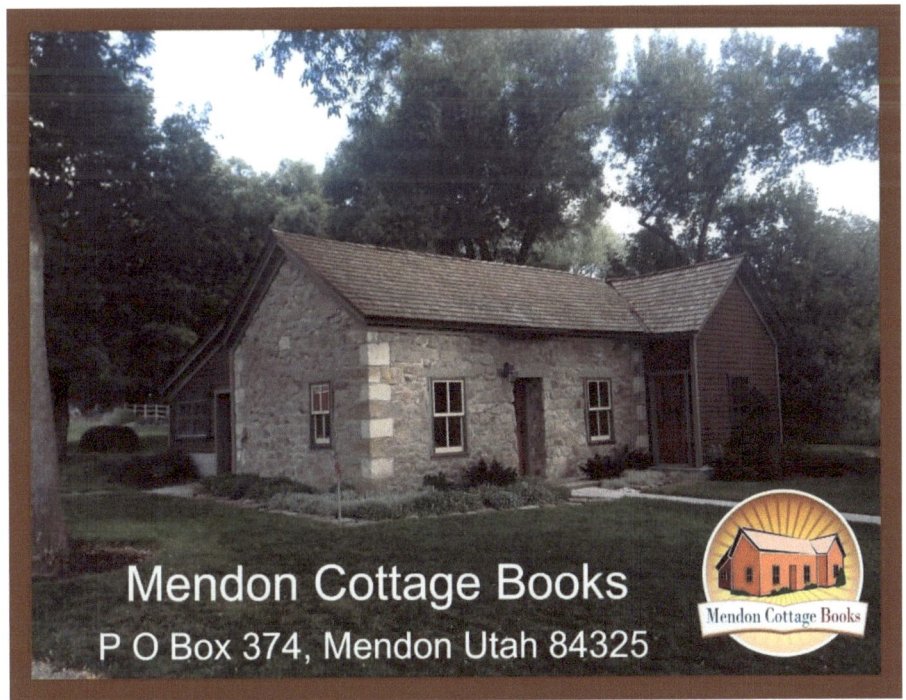

Mendon Cottage Books

P O Box 374, Mendon Utah 84325